1

ORNISH DIET

Cookbook

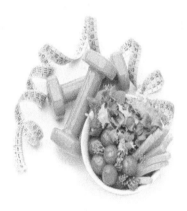

"Reversing Your Heart Disease: Wholesome Recipes for a Healthy Vibrant Life to Lose Weight with the Ornish Diet".

CURNOW K. RIVERS

DISCLAIMER NOTICE:
Please keep in mind that the information in this booklet is solely for educational and entertainment purposes. Every effort has been made to offer complete, accurate, and up-to-date information. There are no express or implied guarantees of any kind. Readers understand that the author is not providing legal, financial, medical, or other professional advice. By reading this document, the reader accepts that we will not be held liable for any losses, direct or indirect, suffered as a result of the use of the information included herein, including but not limited to, errors, omissions, or inaccuracies.

Table of contents

INTRODUCTION   5

CHAPTER 1   7

UNDERSTANDING THE ORNISH DIET   7

CAUSES OF THE ORNISH DIET   7

BENEFITS   8

FOODS TO CONSUME ON THE ORNISH DIET   10

FOODS TO AVOID ON THE ORNISH DIET   11

CHAPTER 2   13

BREAKFAST RECIPES   13

CHAPTER 3   27

LUNCH RECIPES   27

CHAPTER 4   45

DINNER RECIPES   45

CHAPTER 5   61

SNACKS AND SMOOTHIE   61

CONCLUSION   73

14 DAY MEAL PLAN   74

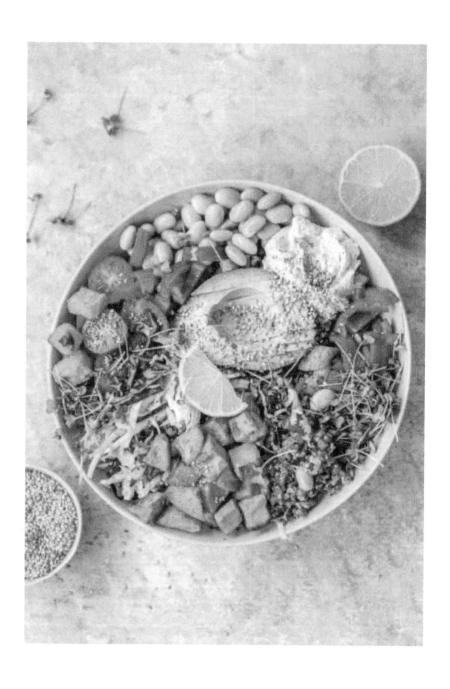

INTRODUCTION

Katie's Inspirational Journey to Vibrant Health and the Ornish Diet: A Path to Transformation
In her desperation to get past her health issues, Katie discovered herself at a crossroads. She was troubled by her extra weight, high cholesterol, and constant lack of energy. She then learned about the Ornish Diet's ability to transform her life—a comprehensive approach to diet and lifestyle.

Katie submerged herself in the Ornish Diet with a relentless determination. This ground-breaking regimen, created by recognized expert Dr. Dean Ornish, emphasizes entire, plant-based diets and holistic well-being. Katie understood that this wasn't just another temporary fix, but rather a sign of optimism for long-term energy and improved health.

Katie stocked her kitchen with colorful fruits, crisp veggies, healthy whole grains, and protein-packed legumes in accordance with the tenets of the Ornish Diet. As she bravely experimented with vivid ingredients, each meal evolved into a celebration of tastes and nourishment.

Months followed weeks, and Katie's dedication was rewarded. A leaner, more vivacious body was revealed as the extra weight disappeared.

However, Katie underwent a tremendous inner shift that went far beyond the physical changes.

Her confidence grew, her energy levels skyrocketed, and she exuded a glowing sense of well-being.

Katie's extraordinary experience served as evidence of the Ornish Diet's capacity for transformation. She was moved to share her tale and the amazing recipes that helped her transformation after being inspired by her personal achievement. As a result, the Ornish Diet Cookbook was created, serving as proof of the effectiveness of clean, plant-based meals in reviving the body, the heart, and the spirit.

Katie's tale serves as motivation for everyone who is dealing with comparable difficulties. It emphasizes the extraordinary tenacity of the human soul and the profound influence of selecting a route lined with nourishing, plant-based food. Her experience serves as a reminder that everyone of us possesses the ability to change the course of our lives and embrace a future filled with thriving health and unlimited vigor.

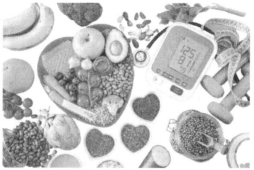

CHAPTER 1

UNDERSTANDING THE ORNISH DIET

The Ornish Diet is a renowned approach to nutrition and lifestyle that focuses on promoting overall health and well-being through a plant-based, low-fat regimen. Developed by Dr. Dean Ornish, a respected expert in preventive medicine, this dietary plan emphasizes the transformative power of whole, natural foods and the avoidance of harmful substances. Let's delve into the causes, benefits, and recommended foods of the Ornish Diet.

CAUSES OF THE ORNISH DIET

The Ornish Diet was born out of the understanding that poor dietary choices and sedentary lifestyles contribute to numerous health problems, including heart disease, obesity, high cholesterol, and hypertension. Dr. Dean Ornish recognized the need for a comprehensive and sustainable approach that addresses these root causes and empowers individuals to take charge of their health.

BENEFITS

The Ornish Diet, developed by Dr. Dean Ornish, offers a multitude of benefits for individuals seeking to improve their health and well-being. This plant-based, low-fat dietary approach has been extensively studied and proven effective in promoting positive changes in various aspects of physical and mental health. Here are some key benefits of the Ornish Diet:

Heart Health: The Ornish Diet has been scientifically proven to reverse the progression of heart disease. By adopting a low-fat, plant-based eating pattern, individuals can lower their cholesterol levels, reduce blood pressure, and improve overall cardiovascular health. This can lead to a decreased risk of heart attacks, strokes, and other cardiovascular complications.

Weight Loss: Following the Ornish Diet can facilitate weight loss and help individuals achieve a healthy body weight. The emphasis on whole, unprocessed foods and the restriction of high-fat and calorie-dense options promotes satiety while reducing overall caloric intake. This can lead to sustainable weight loss and an improvement in body composition.

Diabetes Management: The Ornish Diet can be beneficial for individuals with diabetes or those at risk of developing the condition. By focusing on nutrient-dense, fiber-rich foods and avoiding processed sugars and unhealthy fats, blood sugar levels can be better regulated, and insulin sensitivity can improve. This can aid in managing and preventing type 2 diabetes.

Improved Digestive Health: The emphasis on whole grains, fruits, vegetables, and legumes in the Ornish Diet provides an abundance of dietary fiber. This promotes healthy digestion, aids in maintaining regular bowel movements, and supports a healthy gut microbiome. It can reduce the risk of gastrointestinal disorders such as constipation, diverticulitis, and colon cancer.

Enhanced Mood and Mental Well-being: Research suggests that the Ornish Diet can have positive effects on mental health. The consumption of nutrient-rich foods, particularly those containing omega-3 fatty acids and antioxidants, can support brain health and help alleviate symptoms of depression and anxiety. Additionally, adopting a healthier lifestyle, including regular physical activity, can contribute to improved mental well-being.

Longevity and Disease Prevention: Following the Ornish Diet has been associated with an increased lifespan and a reduced risk of chronic diseases. The emphasis on plant-based foods, which are rich in vitamins, minerals, antioxidants, and phytochemicals, provides the body with essential nutrients and helps protect against various health conditions such as certain cancers, obesity, and metabolic syndrome.

FOODS TO CONSUME ON THE ORNISH DIET

The Ornish Diet places emphasis on whole, unprocessed plant-based foods that are low in fat. These include:

Fruits and Vegetables: Incorporate a variety of colorful fruits and vegetables into your meals, as they are rich in essential vitamins, minerals, and antioxidants.

Whole Grains: Opt for whole grains like brown rice, quinoa, whole wheat bread, and oats, which provide fiber and sustained energy.

Legumes: Include beans, lentils, and chickpeas, as they are excellent sources of plant-based protein and fiber.

Healthy Fats: Consume moderate amounts of healthy fats from sources such as avocados, nuts, and seeds, which provide essential fatty acids.

Non-Fat Dairy or Dairy Alternatives: Choose non-fat dairy products or plant-based alternatives like almond milk or soy milk for added calcium and protein.

FOODS TO AVOID ON THE ORNISH DIET

To adhere to the Ornish Diet, it is recommended to avoid or minimize the intake of the following:

Animal Products: Reduce or eliminate consumption of meat, poultry, fish, and dairy products high in fat.

Processed Foods: Stay away from processed and refined foods such as sugary snacks, refined grains, and packaged meals.

Added Oils: Minimize or avoid the use of oils in cooking, including olive oil, coconut oil, and other high-fat oils.

High-Fat Snacks: Limit consumption of high-fat snacks like chips, fried foods, and pastries.

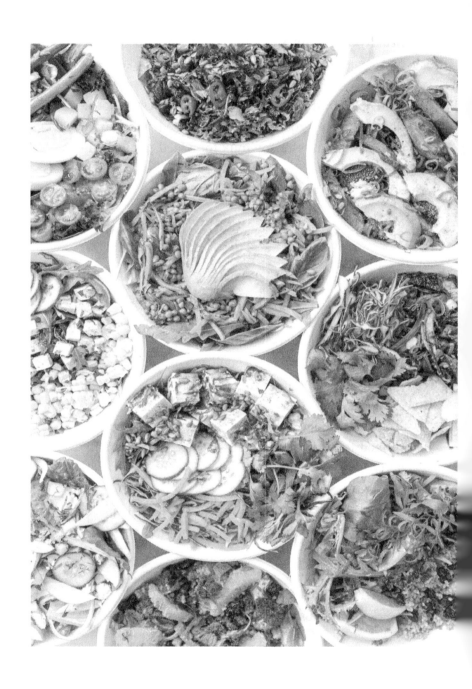

CHAPTER 2

BREAKFAST RECIPES

EGG AND VEGETABLE BREAKFAST WRAP
Ingredients:
Whole wheat tortilla or wrap
Eggs (whites)
Chopped vegetables (e.g., bell peppers, onions, mushrooms)
Fresh herbs (e.g., parsley, basil, cilantro)
Salt and pepper to taste
Cooking spray or olive oil
Instructions:
Heat a non-stick skillet over medium heat and coat with cooking spray or a small amount of olive oil.
Whisk the eggs in a bowl and season with salt and pepper.
Add the chopped vegetables to the skillet and sauté until softened.
Pour the whisked eggs over the vegetables and cook until the eggs are set.
Sprinkle fresh herbs on top for added flavor.
Place the cooked eggs and vegetables in a whole wheat tortilla or wrap.
Roll it up and serve as a satisfying breakfast wrap.

SPINACH AND MUSHROOM EGG WHITE OMELET

Ingredients:
Egg whites from 3 large eggs
Handful of fresh spinach leaves
Sliced mushrooms
Chopped onions
Chopped bell peppers
Salt and pepper to taste
Olive oil or cooking spray

Instructions:
Heat a non-stick skillet over medium heat and coat with olive oil or cooking spray.
Sauté the chopped onions, bell peppers, and mushrooms until softened.
Add the fresh spinach leaves to the skillet and cook until wilted.
In a separate bowl, whisk the egg whites until frothy.
Pour the whisked egg whites over the sautéed vegetables in the skillet.
Season with salt and pepper to taste.
Cook until the egg whites are set and no longer runny.
Carefully fold the omelette in half and slide onto a plate.
Serve with a side of whole grain toast or a mixed greens salad.

GREEK YOGURT PARFAIT
Ingredients:
Greek yogurt (plain or low-fat)
Mixed berries (strawberries, blueberries, raspberries)
Almonds or walnuts (chopped)
Honey or maple syrup (optional for sweetness)
Instructions:
In a glass or bowl, layer Greek yogurt, mixed berries, and chopped nuts.
Repeat the layers until the container is filled.
Drizzle with honey or maple syrup for added sweetness, if desired.
Enjoy the parfait as a protein-packed and antioxidant-rich breakfast option.

QUINOA BREAKFAST BOWL
Ingredients:
Cooked quinoa
Fresh fruits (e.g., sliced banana, diced apple, pomegranate seeds)
Unsweetened almond milk (or any non-dairy milk)
Cinnamon powder
Chia seeds or flaxseeds
Honey or maple syrup for sweetness (optional)
Instructions:

In a bowl, combine cooked quinoa, fresh fruits, a splash of almond milk, a sprinkle of cinnamon powder, and a spoonful of chia seeds or flaxseeds. Mix well until all ingredients are evenly distributed. Sweeten with honey or maple syrup, if desired. Enjoy the nutritious and filling quinoa breakfast bowl.

WHOLE GRAIN OATMEAL WITH BERRIES AND ALMONDS

Ingredients:
1/2 cup whole grain oats
1 cup water or milk (dairy or plant-based)
1/4 teaspoon cinnamon
1/4 teaspoon vanilla extract
1/4 cup mixed berries (such as blueberries, strawberries, raspberries)
1 tablespoon sliced almonds
Optional toppings: honey or maple syrup, chia seeds, additional fruits

Instructions:
In a saucepan, bring the water or milk to a boil over medium heat.
Add the whole grain oats, cinnamon, and vanilla extract to the saucepan.
Stir well and reduce the heat to low.
Cook the oats according to the package instructions, usually for about 5-7 minutes, stirring occasionally.

Once the oats are cooked and have reached your desired consistency, remove the saucepan from the heat.
Transfer the oatmeal to a serving bowl.
Top the oatmeal with the mixed berries and sliced almonds.
Drizzle with honey or maple syrup if desired.
Optional: Sprinkle with chia seeds for added nutritional benefits.
Serve the whole grain oatmeal with berries and almonds hot, and garnish with additional fruits if desired.

SWEET POTATO AND EGG HASH
Ingredients:
Sweet potatoes (peeled and diced)
Chopped onions
Bell peppers (sliced)
Eggs (whites)
Cooking spray
Salt, pepper, and paprika to taste
Fresh parsley (chopped for garnish)
Instructions:
Heat cooking spray in a skillet over medium heat.
Add the diced sweet potatoes, chopped onions, and sliced bell peppers to the skillet.
Sauté until the sweet potatoes are cooked through and slightly crispy.

Make small wells in the hash mixture and pour the egg whites into them.

Season with salt, pepper, and paprika.

Cover the skillet and cook until the eggs are done to your liking.

Garnish with fresh parsley before serving.

SCRAMBLED EGG WHITES WRAP

Ingredients:

4 egg whites

Salt and pepper to taste

Whole grain wrap or tortilla

Spinach leaves

Sliced tomatoes

Sliced avocado

Instructions:

In a bowl, whisk the egg whites until frothy. Season with salt and pepper.

Heat a non-stick skillet over medium heat and pour in the egg whites.

Cook, stirring gently, until the egg whites are fully cooked and scrambled.

Warm the whole grain wrap or tortilla in a separate skillet or microwave.

Place the scrambled egg whites, spinach leaves, sliced tomatoes, and sliced avocado on the wrap.

Roll up the wrap, tucking in the sides, to create a delicious breakfast wrap.

Cut in half and serve.

APPLE CINNAMON QUINOA PORRIDGE
Ingredients:
1/2 cup quinoa, rinsed
1 cup water
1 cup unsweetened almond milk (or any preferred milk)
1 apple, cored and diced
1 tablespoon honey or maple syrup
1/2 teaspoon cinnamon
1/4 teaspoon vanilla extract
Instructions:
In a saucepan, combine the rinsed quinoa, water, and almond milk.
Bring the mixture to a boil over medium heat.
Reduce the heat to low, cover the saucepan, and simmer for 15-20 minutes or until the quinoa is tender and the liquid is absorbed.
Stir in the diced apple, honey or maple syrup, cinnamon, and vanilla extract.
Continue cooking for an additional 2-3 minutes until the apple is softened.
Remove the saucepan from the heat.
Serve the apple cinnamon quinoa porridge hot in bowls.
Enjoy.

FILL-ME-UP SMOOTHIE
Ingredients:
1 medium banana, peeled and chopped

1/2 cup cooked quinoa
1/2 cup Greek yogurt
1/2 cup unsweetened almond milk
1/4 tsp cinnamon
1/4 tsp vanilla extract
Instructions:
Add all the ingredients into a blender.
Blend until smooth and creamy.
Taste and adjust sweetness as desired.
Serve immediately and enjoy.

FRESH GARDEN
Ingredients:
1 cup chopped kale
1 medium cucumber, chopped
1/2 medium avocado, peeled and pitted
1 medium green apple, cored and chopped
1/2 medium lime, juiced
1/2 cup water
Instructions:
Add all the ingredients into a blender.
Blend until smooth and creamy.
Taste and adjust sweetness as desired.
Serve immediately and enjoy.

LEAN GREENIE
Ingredients:
1 cup chopped kale
1 medium green apple, cored and chopped
1 medium cucumber, chopped
1/2 medium avocado, peeled and pitted
1/2 cup coconut water
1/2 lemon, juiced
Instructions:
Add all the ingredients into a blender.
Blend until smooth and creamy.
Taste and adjust sweetness as desired.
Serve immediately and enjoy.

LETTUCE & ORANGE SMOOTHIE
Ingredients:
1 cup lettuce leaves
1 orange, peeled and seeded
1 banana
1/2 cup almond milk
1 tablespoon honey
1/2 teaspoon vanilla extract
Instructions:
In a blender, add lettuce leaves, orange, banana, almond milk, honey, and vanilla extract.
Blend the mixture until smooth.
Pour into a glass and enjoy.

BANANA PANCAKES
Ingredients:
2 ripe bananas, mashed
2 eggs
1/4 teaspoon of baking powder
1/4 teaspoon of cinnamon
Pinch of salt
Butter or cooking spray, for greasing the pan
Instructions:
In a medium-sized bowl, whisk together the mashed bananas and eggs until well combined.
Stir in the baking powder, cinnamon, and pinch of salt.
Heat a large nonstick skillet or griddle over medium-high heat.
Grease the skillet or griddle with butter or cooking spray.
Pour about 1/4 cup of the pancake batter onto the hot skillet or griddle.
Cook the pancake for 2-3 minutes, or until bubbles start to form on the surface.
Flip the pancake and cook for an additional 1-2 minutes, or until golden brown on both sides.
Repeat with the remaining pancake batter.
Serve the banana pancakes with your favorite toppings, such as fresh fruit, yogurt, or maple syrup.

TOFU SCRAMBLE WITH VEGETABLES
Ingredients:
1 tablespoon olive oil
½ block of firm tofu, crumbled
1 small onion, diced
1 small red bell pepper, diced
1 small zucchini, diced
1 cup spinach leaves
1 teaspoon turmeric powder
Salt and pepper to taste
Fresh parsley for garnish
Instructions:
Heat olive oil in a skillet over medium heat.
Add the crumbled tofu and sauté for 2-3 minutes.
Stir in the diced onion, red bell pepper, and zucchini. Cook until the vegetables are tender.
Add the spinach leaves and cook until wilted.
Sprinkle turmeric powder, salt, and pepper over the mixture. Stir well to combine.
Remove from heat and garnish with fresh parsley before serving.

KALE & QUINOA BREAKFAST BOWL
Ingredients:
1 cup cooked quinoa
Kale leaves (chopped)
Cherry tomatoes (halved)
Sliced cucumber
Sliced avocado

Hard-boiled egg (sliced egg whites)
Lemon juice
Olive oil
Salt and pepper to taste
Optional toppings: feta cheese, pumpkin seeds, or sunflower seeds

Instructions:
In a bowl, combine the cooked quinoa, chopped kale leaves, cherry tomatoes, sliced cucumber, sliced avocado, and sliced hard-boiled egg whites. Drizzle with lemon juice and olive oil. Season with salt and pepper. Toss well to combine all the ingredients. Optional: Sprinkle with little feta cheese, pumpkin seeds, or sunflower seeds for added flavor and texture. Serve.

POMEGRANATE MINT SMOOTHIE

Ingredients:
1 cup pomegranate seeds
1 frozen banana
1 cup unsweetened almond milk (or any non-dairy milk)
5-6 fresh mint leaves
1 tablespoon honey or maple syrup (optional)
Ice cubes (optional)

Instructions:

In a blender, combine the pomegranate seeds, frozen banana, almond milk, fresh mint leaves, and sweetener (if desired).
Blend on high speed until smooth and creamy.
If desired, add a few ice cubes and blend again to make the smoothie colder and thicker.
Taste the smoothie and adjust the sweetness or mint flavor according to your preference.
Pour the Pomegranate Mint Smoothie into a glass.

OATMEAL MUFFINS
Ingredients:
1 1/2 cups all-purpose flour
1 cup old-fashioned rolled oats
1/2 cup brown sugar
2 tsp baking powder
1/2 tsp baking soda
1/2 tsp salt
1 cup milk
1/4 cup vegetable oil
1 egg (whites)
1 tsp vanilla extract
1/4 cup blueberries (optional)
Instructions:
Preheat the oven to 375°F.
In a large bowl, whisk together flour, rolled oats, brown sugar, baking powder, baking soda, and salt.
In a separate bowl, whisk together milk, vegetable oil, egg whites and vanilla extract.

Pour wet ingredients into dry ingredients, add your berries and mix until just combined.

Pour batter into lined muffin tins, filling each cup about 3/4 full.

Bake for 20-25 minutes, until muffins are golden brown and a toothpick inserted into the center comes out clean.

Allow muffins to cool in the tin for 5 minutes before removing and transferring to a wire rack to cool completely.

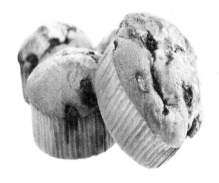

CHAPTER 3

LUNCH RECIPES

VEGGIE AND HUMMUS SANDWICH
Ingredients:
2 slices whole-grain bread
2 tablespoons hummus (flavor of your choice)
1/4 mashed avocado
1/4 cup sliced cucumber
1/4 cup sliced bell peppers (any color)
1/4 cup baby spinach or mixed greens
2-3 slices tomato
2-3 slices red onion
Sprouts (optional)
Salt and pepper to taste
Instructions:
Spread hummus evenly on one slice of bread and the avocado on the other slice.
Layer cucumber slices, bell peppers, baby spinach or mixed greens, tomato slices, red onion slices, and sprouts (if using) on top of the hummus.
Sprinkle with salt and pepper to taste.
Place the second slice of bread on top.
Cut the sandwich in half if desired.
Serve and enjoy

STUFFED BELL PEPPERS WITH GROUND BEEF AND RICE

Ingredients:
4 bell peppers (any color)
1 pound ground beef
1 cup cooked rice
1 small onion, diced
2 cloves garlic, minced
1 can diced tomatoes
1 teaspoon dried oregano
1 teaspoon dried basil
Salt and pepper to taste
Shredded cheese (optional, for topping)

Instructions:
Preheat the oven to 375°F (190°C). Cut off the tops of the bell peppers and remove the seeds and membranes.

In a large skillet, cook the ground beef over medium heat until browned. Drain any excess fat.

Add the diced onion and minced garlic to the skillet and cook until the onion is softened.

Stir in the cooked rice, diced tomatoes (with juices), dried oregano, dried basil, salt, and pepper. Cook for a few minutes to allow the flavors to meld together.

Stuff the bell peppers with the beef and rice mixture and place them in a baking dish.

If desired, sprinkle shredded cheese on top of the stuffed bell peppers.

Bake in the preheated oven for about 25-30 minutes, or until the bell peppers are tender and the filling is heated through. Remove from the oven and let cool slightly before serving.

BROWN RICE AND VEGETABLE STIR-FRY WITH TOFU

Ingredients:

1 package firm tofu, drained and cubed
2 cups mixed vegetables (such as bell peppers, broccoli, mushrooms, snow peas)
2 cloves garlic, minced
2 tablespoons low-sodium soy sauce
1 tablespoon hoisin sauce
1 tablespoon sesame oil
1 tablespoon olive oil
Cooked brown rice for serving

Instructions:

Heat olive oil in a large skillet or wok over medium-high heat.

Add minced garlic to the skillet and stir-fry for about 1 minute until fragrant.

Add the tofu cubes to the skillet and cook for 4-5 minutes until they are golden brown on all sides. Remove the tofu from the skillet and set aside.

In the same skillet, add the mixed vegetables and stir-fry for about 5-7 minutes until they are crisp-tender.

Return the cooked tofu to the skillet with the vegetables.

In a small bowl, whisk together the soy sauce

LENTIL AND VEGETABLE SOUP WITH WHOLE GRAIN BREAD

Ingredients:

1 cup dried lentils
1 tablespoon olive oil
1 onion, diced
2 carrots, diced
2 celery stalks, diced
2 cloves garlic, minced
1 teaspoon dried thyme
1 teaspoon dried oregano
4 cups vegetable broth
2 cups water
1 bay leaf
Salt and pepper to taste
Fresh parsley for garnish
Whole grain bread for serving

Instructions:

Rinse the dried lentils under cold water and set them aside.

Heat the olive oil in a large pot over medium heat.

Add the diced onion, carrots, celery, and minced garlic to the pot. Sauté until the vegetables start to soften.

Stir in the dried thyme and dried oregano, and cook for another minute to release their flavors. Add the rinsed lentils, vegetable broth, water, bay leaf, salt, and pepper to the pot. Stir well to combine.

Bring the soup to a boil, then reduce the heat to low and let it simmer for about 30-40 minutes, or until the lentils are tender.

Remove the bay leaf and taste the soup. Adjust the seasonings if needed.

Serve the lentil and vegetable soup hot, garnished with fresh parsley. Pair it with whole grain bread for a complete and satisfying meal.

BLACK BEAN CHILI & SWEET POTATO

Ingredients:
1 tablespoon olive oil
1 onion, diced
2 cloves garlic, minced
1 sweet potato, peeled and diced
1 red bell pepper, diced
1 green bell pepper, diced
1 can (15 ounces) black beans, rinsed and drained
1 can (14 ounces) diced tomatoes
1 cup vegetable broth
1 tablespoon chili powder
1 teaspoon cumin
1/2 teaspoon smoked paprika
Salt and pepper to taste

Fresh chopped cilantro for garnish
Instructions:
Heat the olive oil in a large pot or Dutch oven over medium heat.

Add the diced onion and minced garlic to the pot. Sauté for 2-3 minutes until the onion becomes translucent and the garlic is fragrant.

Add the diced sweet potato, red bell pepper, and green bell pepper to the pot. Cook for 5 minutes, stirring occasionally, until the vegetables begin to soften.

Add the black beans, diced tomatoes, vegetable broth, chili powder, cumin, smoked paprika, salt, and pepper to the pot. Stir well to combine.

Bring the mixture to a boil, then reduce the heat to low. Cover the pot and simmer for 20-25 minutes, or until the sweet potatoes are tender.

Taste and adjust the seasonings as needed.

Serve the sweet potato and black bean chili hot, garnished with fresh chopped cilantro.

QUINOA AND VEGETABLE STUFFED BELL PEPPERS
Ingredients:
4 bell peppers (assorted colors)
1 cup cooked quinoa
1 zucchini, diced
1 yellow squash, diced
1 onion, diced

2 cloves garlic, minced
1 cup diced tomatoes
1 teaspoon dried oregano
1 teaspoon dried basil
Salt and pepper to taste
1/4 cup grated Parmesan cheese (optional)
Fresh parsley for garnish

Instructions:

Preheat the oven to 375°F (190°C).

Slice off the tops of the bell peppers and remove the seeds and membranes.

In a large skillet, heat a little bit of olive oil over medium heat.

Add the diced zucchini, yellow squash, onion, and minced garlic to the skillet. Sauté until the vegetables are tender and slightly golden.

Stir in the cooked quinoa, diced tomatoes, dried oregano, dried basil, salt, and pepper. Mix well to combine all the ingredients.

Spoon the quinoa and vegetable mixture into the hollowed-out bell peppers, pressing it down gently.

Sprinkle the grated Parmesan cheese over the stuffed bell peppers if desired.

Place the stuffed bell peppers in a baking dish and cover with foil.

Bake in the preheated oven for about 30-35 minutes, or until the bell peppers are tender and the filling is heated through.

Remove from the oven and garnish with fresh parsley.

Serve the quinoa and vegetable stuffed bell peppers hot as a nutritious and satisfying lunch option.

VEGETABLE AND TOFU CURRY

Ingredients:

1 block firm tofu, drained and cubed
1 tablespoon vegetable oil
1 onion, diced
2 cloves garlic, minced
1 tablespoon grated ginger
2 bell peppers, sliced
1 zucchini, sliced
1 cup cauliflower florets
1 cup broccoli florets
1 can (14 oz) coconut milk
2 tablespoons curry powder
1 teaspoon turmeric
1/2 teaspoon cumin
Salt and pepper to taste
Fresh cilantro for garnish
Cooked brown rice or quinoa for serving

Instructions:

Heat the vegetable oil in a large skillet or wok over medium heat.

Add the diced onion, minced garlic, and grated ginger to the skillet. Sauté until the onion becomes translucent and fragrant.

Add the tofu cubes to the skillet and cook for a few minutes until lightly browned.

Stir in the sliced bell peppers, zucchini, cauliflower florets, and broccoli florets. Cook for another 3-4 minutes until the vegetables start to soften.

In a small bowl, whisk together the coconut milk, curry powder, turmeric, cumin, salt, and pepper.

Pour the coconut milk mixture over the vegetables and tofu in the skillet. Stir well to combine.

Reduce the heat to low, cover the skillet, and let the curry simmer for about 10-12 minutes, stirring occasionally, until the vegetables are tender and the flavors have melded together.

Taste and adjust the seasonings if needed.

Serve the vegetable and tofu curry hot, garnished with fresh cilantro, and accompanied by cooked brown rice or quinoa.

CLASSIC TOMATO AND BASIL SALAD

Ingredients:

4 large ripe tomatoes, sliced

1 cup fresh basil leaves, torn

1 small red onion, thinly sliced

½ cup fresh mozzarella cheese, cubed

2 tablespoons extra virgin olive oil

1 tablespoon balsamic vinegar

Salt and pepper to taste

Instructions:

Arrange the tomato slices on a serving platter or individual plates.
Scatter the torn basil leaves over the tomatoes.
Add the thinly sliced red onion and mozzarella cheese.
In a small bowl, whisk together the olive oil, balsamic vinegar, salt, and pepper.
Drizzle the dressing over the salad.
Serve immediately and enjoy this classic combination

GRILLED TOFU AND VEGETABLE KEBABS WITH BROWN RICE

Ingredients:
1 package firm tofu, drained and cubed
1 zucchini, sliced into rounds
1 yellow squash, sliced into rounds
1 red onion, cut into chunks
1 bell pepper, cut into chunks
2 tablespoons olive oil
2 tablespoons soy sauce
1 tablespoon balsamic vinegar
1 teaspoon dried basil
1 teaspoon dried oregano
Salt and pepper to taste
Cooked brown rice for serving
Instructions:
Preheat the grill to medium heat.

In a large bowl, whisk together olive oil, soy sauce, balsamic vinegar, dried basil, dried oregano, salt, and pepper. Add the cubed tofu, sliced zucchini, sliced yellow squash, onion chunks, and bell pepper chunks to the bowl. Toss to coat the tofu and vegetables in the marinade. Thread the marinated tofu and vegetables onto skewers, alternating between tofu and vegetables. Place the kebabs on the preheated grill and cook for about 10-12 minutes, turning occasionally, until the tofu and vegetables are lightly charred and cooked through. Serve the grilled tofu and vegetable kebabs over cooked brown rice.

LENTIL SOUP WITH CARROTS AND CELERY

Ingredients:
1 cup dried lentils
2 tablespoons olive oil
1 onion, chopped
2 carrots, diced
2 celery stalks, diced
3 cloves garlic, minced
4 cups vegetable broth
1 teaspoon dried thyme
1 bay leaf
Salt and pepper to taste

Fresh parsley for garnish
Instructions:
Rinse the lentils under cold water and set aside.
Heat olive oil in a large pot over medium heat.
Add the chopped onion, carrots, celery, and minced garlic. Sauté until the vegetables are tender.
Add the lentils, vegetable broth, dried thyme, bay leaf, salt, and pepper to the pot.
Bring the mixture to a boil, then reduce the heat and simmer for about 30-40 minutes, or until the lentils are cooked and tender.
Remove the bay leaf and adjust the seasoning if needed.
Serve the lentil soup hot, garnished with fresh parsley.

HERBED SAVORY QUINOA
Ingredients:
1 cup quinoa
2 cups vegetable broth
1 tablespoon olive oil
1 onion, diced
2 cloves garlic, minced
1 teaspoon dried herbs (such as thyme, rosemary, or oregano)
Salt and pepper to taste
Fresh parsley for garnish
Instructions:
Rinse the quinoa under cold water and drain.

In a saucepan, bring the vegetable broth to a boil. Add the quinoa to the boiling broth, cover, and reduce the heat to low. Simmer for about 15-20 minutes or until the quinoa is cooked and the liquid is absorbed. In a separate pan, heat olive oil over medium heat. Sauté the diced onion and minced garlic until fragrant and lightly browned. Add the cooked quinoa to the pan with the sautéed onion and garlic. Season with dried herbs, salt, and pepper. Stir well to combine. Cook for another 2-3 minutes to allow the flavors to meld. Serve the savory herbed quinoa garnished with fresh parsley.

VEGETABLE FRIED CAULIFLOWER RICE
Ingredients:
1 medium head cauliflower, grated or processed into rice-like texture
2 tablespoons olive oil
1 onion, diced
2 carrots, diced
1 red bell pepper, diced
1 cup peas (fresh or frozen)
2 cloves garlic, minced
2 tablespoons low-sodium soy sauce (or tamari for a gluten-free option)

Salt and pepper to taste

Chopped green onions for garnish

Instructions:

Heat olive oil in a large skillet or wok over medium heat.

Add the diced onion, carrots, red bell pepper, peas, and minced garlic to the skillet. Sauté until the vegetables are tender-crisp.

Push the vegetables to one side of the skillet and add the grated cauliflower rice to the other side.

Cook the cauliflower rice for 5-6 minutes, stirring occasionally, until it becomes tender.

Mix the cooked vegetables with the cauliflower rice in the skillet.

Drizzle the low-sodium soy sauce over the mixture and stir well to combine.

Season with salt and pepper according to your taste.

Cook for another 2-3 minutes to allow the flavors to blend.

Serve the vegetable fried cauliflower rice hot, garnished with chopped green onions.

ZUCCHINI NOODLES WITH TOFU AND TOMATO SAUCE

Ingredients:

2 medium zucchinis, spiralized

1 pound tofu, diced into cubes

2 cloves garlic, minced

1 can (14 ounces) diced tomatoes

1 teaspoon dried basil
1 teaspoon dried oregano
Salt and pepper to taste
Fresh basil leaves for garnish
Instructions:
In a large skillet, heat olive oil over medium heat. Add minced garlic and sauté until fragrant. Add the tofu to the skillet and cook for 2-3 minutes on each side until golden brown and cook through. Remove the tofu from the skillet and set aside. In the same skillet, add the diced tomatoes, dried basil, dried oregano, salt, and pepper. Simmer the tomato sauce for about 5 minutes to allow the flavors to meld. Add the spiralized zucchini noodles to the skillet and toss them with the tomato sauce. Cook for 2-3 minutes until the noodles are tender-crisp. Return the cooked tofu to the skillet and toss them with the zucchini noodles and tomato sauce. Serve the zucchini noodles with tofu and tomato sauce in bowls, garnished with fresh basil leaves.

CREAMY SPLIT PEA SOUP
Ingredients:
1 cup split peas, rinsed and drained
1 tablespoon olive oil
1 onion, chopped
2 cloves garlic, minced
2 carrots, diced

2 stalks celery, diced
4 cups vegetable broth
1 teaspoon dried thyme
Salt and pepper to taste
Fresh parsley for garnish
Instructions:
In a large pot, heat the olive oil over medium heat.
Add the chopped onion and minced garlic. Sauté
until the onion becomes translucent and fragrant.
Add the diced carrots and celery to the pot. Cook
until the vegetables are tender.
Add the rinsed split peas, vegetable broth, dried
thyme, salt, and pepper to the pot.
Bring the mixture to a boil, then reduce the heat and
simmer for about 45-60 minutes, or until the split
peas are soft and cooked through.
Use an immersion blender or transfer the soup to a
blender to puree until smooth and creamy.
If needed, return the soup to the pot and heat it
gently before serving.
Garnish with fresh parsley.

CHICKPEAS AND QUINOA SALAD
Ingredients:
1 cup cooked quinoa
1 can chickpeas, rinsed and drained
1 cucumber, diced
1 red bell pepper, diced
1 small red onion, finely chopped

½ cup cherry tomatoes, halved
¼ cup fresh parsley, chopped
¼ cup fresh mint leaves, chopped
Juice of 1 lemon
2 tablespoons extra virgin olive oil
Salt and pepper to taste
Instructions:
In a large mixing bowl, combine the cooked quinoa,
chickpeas, diced cucumber, diced red bell pepper,
chopped red onion, cherry tomatoes, fresh parsley,
and fresh mint leaves.
In a small bowl, whisk together the lemon juice,
extra virgin olive oil, salt, and pepper.
Pour the dressing over the salad and toss well to
coat all the ingredients.
Taste the salad and adjust the seasoning if needed.
Let the salad sit for about 10-15 minutes to allow
the flavors to meld together.
Serve.

MILLET LETTUCE WRAPS
Ingredients:
1 cup cooked millet
1 tablespoon olive oil
1 onion, diced
2 cloves garlic, minced
1 red bell pepper, diced
1 carrot, grated
1 zucchini, diced

1 cup mushrooms, sliced
1 tablespoon soy sauce (or tamari for a gluten-free option)
1 tablespoon rice vinegar
Salt and pepper to taste
Lettuce leaves for wrapping
Optional toppings: chopped green onions, sesame seeds

Instructions:

Heat olive oil in a large pan over medium heat.

Add the diced onion and minced garlic. Sauté until fragrant and lightly browned.

Add the red bell pepper, grated carrot, diced zucchini, and sliced mushrooms to the pan. Cook until the vegetables are tender.

Stir in the cooked millet and season with soy sauce, rice vinegar, salt, and pepper. Mix well to combine.

Remove the pan from heat and let the mixture cool slightly.

Spoon the millet and vegetable mixture onto lettuce leaves.

Garnish with chopped green onions and sesame seeds, if desired.

Roll up the lettuce leaves to form wraps and secure with toothpicks if needed.

Serve the Millet Lettuce Wraps as a light and flavorful meal.

CHAPTER 4

DINNER RECIPES

LENTIL AND VEGETABLE TACOS WITH WHOLE WHEAT TORTILLAS

Ingredients:
1 cup cooked lentils
1 tablespoon olive oil
1 onion, diced
2 cloves garlic, minced
1 red bell pepper, diced
1 zucchini, diced
1 cup corn kernels (fresh or frozen)
1 teaspoon ground cumin
1 teaspoon chili powder
Salt and pepper to taste
Whole wheat tortillas
Toppings: diced tomatoes, shredded lettuce, sliced avocado, salsa, Greek yogurt (optional)

Instructions:
Olive oil should be warmed in a big pan over medium heat.

Add the minced garlic and onion. Cook until aromatic and just beginning to brown.

To the pan, add the diced red bell pepper, zucchini, and corn. Cook the vegetables until they are soft.

Add the cooked lentils together with the salt, pepper, ground cumin, and chili powder. Heat thoroughly after combining thoroughly.

The whole wheat tortillas can be warmed in the oven or a dry skillet.

Each tortilla should have a spoonful of the lentil and veggie mixture on it.

Add desired toppings, such as Greek yogurt, salsa, sliced avocado, chopped tomatoes, and lettuce.

To make tacos, fold the tortillas over the filling.

Serve the tacos with lentils and vegetables.

BLACK BEANS WITH QUINOA STUFFED PEPPERS CORN

Ingredients:

4 bell peppers (any color)

1 cup cooked quinoa

1 can black beans, rinsed and drained

1 cup corn kernels (fresh or frozen)

1 small onion, diced

2 cloves garlic, minced

1 teaspoon ground cumin

1 teaspoon chili powder

Salt and pepper to taste

1 cup shredded cheese (cheddar)

Fresh cilantro for garnish

Instructions:

Set the oven's temperature to 375°F (190°C). Butter a baking pan.

Remove the bell peppers' tops, then scoop out the seeds and membranes.

Cooked quinoa, black beans, corn, onion, garlic, cumin, chili powder, salt, and pepper should all be combined in a sizable mixing dish. Mix thoroughly. Fill every bell pepper to the top with the quinoa mixture.

In the baking dish that has been buttered, put the stuffed peppers. Wrap with foil.

Bake the peppers for 25 to 30 minutes, or until they are soft.

Shredded cheese is then added to the peppers after the foil has been removed.

If the cheese isn't melted and bubbling after 5 minutes, put the baking dish back in the oven.

Add fresh cilantro as a garnish.

LENTIL SOUP
Ingredients:
1 cup dried lentils (any variety)
1 tablespoon olive oil
1 onion, chopped
2 cloves garlic, minced
2 carrots, diced
2 celery stalks, diced
4 cups vegetable broth
1 can diced tomatoes
1 teaspoon dried thyme
Salt and pepper to taste

Fresh parsley for garnish
Instructions:
Drain the lentils after giving them a cold water rinse.
Olive oil should be heated in a sizable pot over medium heat.
Add the minced garlic and onion, both chopped.
The onion should be sautéed until aromatic and transparent.
To the pot, add the diced celery and carrots. Cook the vegetables just until they start to soften.
To the pot, add the lentils, vegetable broth, diced tomatoes, salt, pepper, and any additional liquids.
To blend, thoroughly stir.
When the lentils are ready, simmer the mixture for around 25 to 30 minutes after bringing it to a boil.
If necessary, adjust the seasoning.
Into bowls, ladle the lentil soup.
Add fresh parsley as a garnish.

ROASTED CORN SOUP
Ingredients:
4 ears of corn
1 tablespoon olive oil
1 onion, chopped
2 cloves garlic, minced
4 cups vegetable broth
1 teaspoon ground cumin
1 teaspoon smoked paprika

Salt and pepper to taste
Fresh cilantro for garnish
Instructions:
Set the oven's temperature to 400°F (200°C).
On a baking sheet, arrange the corn ears and sprinkle with olive oil. Add salt and pepper to taste. The corn should be roasted in the preheated oven for 20 to 25 minutes, or until the kernels are golden and just beginning to sear.
Corn should be taken out of the oven to cool. Cut the kernels off the cobs once they have cooled.
Olive oil is heated over medium heat in a big pot.
Add the minced garlic and onion, both chopped. The onion should be sautéed until aromatic and transparent.
To intensify the tastes, add the roasted corn kernels to the pot and cook for a short while.
Bring the mixture to a boil after adding the veggie broth. Simmer for ten to fifteen minutes on low heat.
Cumin and smoked paprika should be stirred in. Add pepper and salt to taste when seasoning.
Pour the soup into a blender or use an immersion blender to purée it until smooth.
Put the soup back in the pot and heat it slowly.
Pour bowls with the roasted corn soup.
Garnish with fresh cilantro.

ASPARAGUS CREAMY SOUP
Ingredients:
1 lb (450g) asparagus, trimmed and chopped
1 tablespoon olive oil
1 onion, chopped
2 cloves garlic, minced
4 cups vegetable broth
1 cup coconut milk
Salt and pepper to taste
Fresh chives for garnish
Instructions:
Over medium heat, warm the olive oil in a big pot.
Add the minced garlic and onion, which have been chopped. The onion should be sautéed until it turns transparent and smells good.
Asparagus should be added to the pot and cooked for a few minutes until slightly mushy.
Add the vegetable broth, then bring the mixture to a boil. Once the asparagus is cooked, turn down the heat and let it simmer for 15 to 20 minutes.
Pour the soup into a blender or use an immersion blender to purée it until smooth.
Add the coconut milk to the soup before bringing it back to a simmer. Warm up the soup thoroughly over a low heat.
Add pepper and salt to taste.
Pour the creamy asparagus soup into dishes.
Add some fresh parsley as a garnish.

EASY VEGGIE NOODLE BOWLS
Ingredients:
8 ounces (225g) noodles (such as rice noodles or soba noodles)
2 tablespoons soy sauce
1 tablespoon sesame oil
1 tablespoon rice vinegar
1 teaspoon honey or maple syrup
1 teaspoon grated ginger
1 clove garlic, minced
1 cup mixed vegetables (such as bell peppers, carrots, snow peas)
1 cup bean sprouts
2 green onions, sliced
Sesame seeds for garnish
Toppings: sliced tofu
Instructions:
Noodles should be cooked as directed on the packaging. Drain, then set apart.

To create the sauce, combine the soy sauce, sesame oil, rice vinegar, honey or maple syrup, grated ginger, and chopped garlic in a small bowl and whisk until well combined.

A large pan or wok should be heated over medium heat with a little oil.

When the mixed veggies have softened, add them to the pan and stir-fry for a short while.

For one more minute, stir-fry the green onions and bean sprouts in the pan.

Pour the sauce over the cooked noodles after adding them to the pan. Toss everything together to evenly distribute the sauce and coat the noodles and vegetables.

Cook the noodles for a further 1-2 minutes, or until they are thoroughly warm.

Remove from heat and divide the noodle-veggie mixture into bowls.

Garnish with sesame seeds.

If desired, add your choice of toppings such as sliced tofu.

GREEN BEANS AND MUSHROOMS STIR-FRY

Ingredients:

1 lb (450g) green beans, ends trimmed

8 ounces (225g) mushrooms, sliced

2 tablespoons soy sauce

1 tablespoon sesame oil

2 cloves garlic, minced

1 teaspoon grated ginger

1 tablespoon olive oil

Salt and pepper to taste

Sesame seeds for garnish

Instructions:

Boil some salted water in a pot. Green beans should be crisp-tender after about 2-3 minutes of cooking after being added. Drain, then set apart.

To prepare the sauce, combine the soy sauce, sesame oil, minced garlic, and grated ginger in a small bowl.

In a sizable skillet or wok, heat the olive oil over medium-high heat.

Sliced mushrooms should be added to the skillet and stir-fried for about 5 minutes, or until brown and just softened.

Green beans that have been blanched should be added to the skillet and stir-fried for an additional 2 to 3 minutes.

The vegetables should be covered equally with the sauce after being poured over them.

To fully heat and enable the flavors to meld, cook for a further minute.

Season with salt and pepper to taste.

Remove from heat and sprinkle with sesame seeds.

TOFU AND VEGETABLE SOUP
Ingredients:
Firm tofu, cubed
Mixed vegetables (such as carrots, broccoli, bell peppers), chopped
Mushroom, chopped
Onion, chopped
Garlic cloves, minced
Vegetable broth
Soy sauce (or tamari for gluten-free option)
Sesame oil

Ginger, grated
Green onions, sliced
Salt and pepper to taste
Olive oil

Instructions:

In a large pot, heat some olive oil over medium heat. Add the chopped onion and minced garlic cloves. Sauté until the onion becomes translucent and the garlic becomes fragrant.

Add the mixed vegetables and mushrooms to the pot and sauté for a few minutes until they begin to soften.

Pour in enough vegetable broth to cover the vegetables. Bring the mixture to a boil, then reduce the heat and let it simmer until the vegetables are tender.

Add the cubed tofu to a non stick pot and fry little on each sides

Add the lightly fried tofu and let it simmer for a few more minutes to heat through.

Stir in soy sauce, sesame oil, and grated ginger.

Season with salt and pepper to taste.

Ladle the soup into bowls and garnish with sliced green onions.

Serve the tofu and vegetable soup hot. Enjoy!

CARROT SOUP

Ingredients:

Carrots, peeled and chopped
Onion, chopped
Garlic cloves, minced
Vegetable broth
Fresh ginger, grated (optional)
Ground cumin
Ground coriander
Salt and pepper to taste
Olive oil
Fresh cilantro or parsley for garnish (optional)

Instructions:

In a large pot, heat some olive oil over medium heat. Add the chopped onion and minced garlic cloves. Sauté until the onion becomes translucent and the garlic becomes fragrant.

Add the chopped carrots to the pot and cook for a few minutes, stirring occasionally.

Pour in enough vegetable broth to cover the carrots. Bring the mixture to a boil, then reduce the heat and let it simmer until the carrots are tender.

If desired, add grated ginger, ground cumin, and ground coriander to the pot for added flavor. Stir well.

Using an immersion blender or a regular blender, blend the soup until smooth and creamy.

Return the soup to the pot and season with salt and pepper to taste.

Heat the soup over low heat until it is warmed through.

Serve the carrot soup hot, garnished with fresh cilantro or parsley if desired.

BUCKWHEAT WITH MUSHROOMS & GREEN ONION

Ingredients:

1 cup buckwheat groats

2 cups vegetable broth

1 tablespoon olive oil

8 ounces (225g) mushrooms, sliced

2 green onions, sliced

2 cloves garlic, minced

Salt and pepper to taste

Fresh parsley for garnish

Instructions:

Buckwheat groats should be rinsed with cold water.

Activate the boiling process of the vegetable broth in a medium pot. Turn down the heat, then stir in the groats of washed buckwheat. For around 15-20 minutes, or when the buckwheat is soft and the liquid is absorbed, cover and simmer the dish.

Olive oil should be heated in a sizable skillet over medium heat while the buckwheat is cooking.

Add the mushroom slices and cook them for 5 to 7 minutes, or until they are golden brown and soft.

Add the minced garlic and green onions after mixing. Cook for a further two minutes.

To taste, add salt and pepper to the food. With a fork, fluff the cooked buckwheat before adding it to the skillet with the mushrooms and green onions. Mix well to combine. Cook for another 2-3 minutes to allow the flavors to meld together. Remove from heat and garnish with fresh parsley.

ZUCCHINI LINGUINI WITH SPINACH AND BASIL PESTO

Ingredients:
4 medium zucchinis
2 cups fresh spinach leaves
1 cup fresh basil leaves
1/2 cup grated Parmesan cheese
1/4 cup pine nuts
2 cloves garlic, minced
1/4 cup olive oil
Juice of 1 lemon
Salt and pepper to taste
Cherry tomatoes for garnish (optional)
Fresh basil leaves for garnish

Instructions:
Slice the zucchinis into long, thin strips that resemble pasta using a spiralizer or a julienne peeler to make zucchini linguini.

Put the zucchini linguini in a sieve with a little salt on top. To release extra moisture, let them sit for around 10 minutes. Squeeze out any liquid that is still present after that.

Combine the spinach, basil, Parmesan cheese, pine nuts, garlic powder, olive oil, and lemon juice in a food processor. Process until well-combined and fluid.

To taste, add salt and pepper to the pesto.

A light drizzle of olive oil should be heated in a big skillet over medium heat.

To the skillet, add the zucchini linguini, and cook for 2 to 3 minutes, or until just tender.

After taking the skillet off the heat, combine the zucchini linguini with the spinach and basil pesto. Toss everything together until the pesto is uniformly distributed over the linguini.

Serve and garnish with cherry tomatoes and fresh basil leaves, if desired.

REFRESHING SUMMER ROLLS
Ingredients:
8 rice paper wrappers
8 lettuce leaves
1 cup cooked rice vermicelli noodles
1 cup julienned carrots
1 cup julienned cucumbers
1 cup thinly sliced bell peppers
1 cup fresh mint leaves
1 cup fresh cilantro leaves
1/2 cup chopped peanuts (optional)

Hoisin sauce or peanut sauce for dipping
Instructions:
Make a shallow dish and fill it with warm water. One rice paper wrapper should be briefly dipped into the water to make it more malleable and soft. Transferring the softened rice paper wrapper onto a spotless, level surface requires caution. Lay a lettuce leaf on the rice paper wrapper's bottom half. The lettuce leaf should be covered with a thin layer of rice vermicelli noodles. On top of the noodles, scatter some of the julienned bell peppers, carrots, cucumbers, mint, and cilantro. To give the vegetables some crunch, if desired, scatter some chopped peanuts on top. To enclose the filling, fold the sides of the rice paper wrapper inward and then tightly roll it up from the bottom. Utilizing the remaining materials, repeat this procedure. If preferred, cut the summer rolls in half diagonally and offer hoisin or peanut sauce for dipping.

RAW ZUCCHINI AND TOMATO LASAGNA
Ingredients:
3 medium zucchinis
4 large tomatoes
1 cup fresh basil leaves
1 cup raw cashews
1/4 cup nutritional yeast

2 cloves garlic

Juice of 1 lemon

Salt and pepper to taste

Extra virgin olive oil for drizzling

Instructions:

Round out the tomatoes and zucchinis with a knife. Combine the basil leaves, cashews, nutritional yeast, garlic cloves, lemon juice, salt, and pepper in a food processor. The mixture should be processed until it resembles creamy pesto.

Start arranging the zucchini rounds in a rectangle baking dish as the foundation.

Over the rounds of zucchini, apply a layer of the smooth basil pesto.

On top of the pesto, arrange a layer of tomato rounds.

Till you run out of ingredients, keep layering alternately zucchini rounds, basil pesto rounds, and tomato rounds.

On top of the last layer, drizzle some extra virgin olive oil.

Cover the baking dish with plastic wrap and refrigerate for at least 2 hours to allow the flavors to meld and the lasagna to set.

Remove the lasagna from the refrigerator and slice it into squares or rectangles.

CHAPTER 5

SNACKS AND SMOOTHIE

+DESSERT

GUACAMOLE WITH CELERY STICKS

Ingredients:
2 ripe avocados, peeled and pitted
1 small tomato, seeded and diced
1/4 red onion, diced
1 garlic clove, minced
1 lime, juiced
1/4 tsp sea salt
4 celery stalks, cut into sticks

Instructions:
In a medium bowl, mash the avocados with a fork until they're slightly chunky.
Add the tomato, red onion, garlic, lime juice, and sea salt to the bowl with the avocados and stir until well combined.
Serve the guacamole immediately with the celery sticks for dipping.

CUCUMBER SALAD

Ingredients:
2 large cucumbers, peeled and sliced thinly
1/4 red onion, thinly sliced
1/4 cup chopped fresh dill
1/4 cup white vinegar

1 tablespoon honey
Salt and pepper to taste
Instructions:
In a large bowl, combine the sliced cucumbers, red onion, and chopped dill.
In a separate bowl, whisk together the white vinegar, honey, salt, and pepper until the honey is dissolved.
Pour the dressing over the cucumber mixture and toss to coat.
Chill in the refrigerator for at least 30 minutes before serving.

SPINACH SMOOTHIE
Ingredients:
1 cup spinach leaves
1 banana, peeled and sliced
1/2 cup frozen mango chunks
1/2 cup almond milk
1/2 cup plain Greek yogurt
1 tablespoon honey
1/4 teaspoon vanilla extract
1/4 teaspoon ground cinnamon
Instructions:
Combine all the ingredients in a blender and blend until smooth.
Pour into a glass and enjoy immediately.

KALE SMOOTHIE
Ingredients:
1 cup kale leaves, chopped
1 banana, peeled and sliced
1/2 cup frozen pineapple chunks
1/2 cup coconut water
1/2 cup plain Greek yogurt
1 tablespoon honey
1/4 teaspoon vanilla extract
1/4 teaspoon ground ginger
Instructions:
Combine all the ingredients in a blender and blend
until smooth.
Pour into a glass and enjoy immediately.

CELERY CARROT JUICE
Ingredients:
4 celery stalks
2 large carrots
1/2 inch fresh ginger root
1/2 lemon, juiced
Instructions:
Wash the celery stalks and carrots and cut them into
small pieces.
Peel and cut the ginger root into small pieces.
Pass the celery, carrots, and ginger through a juicer,
collecting the juice in a container.
Stir in the lemon juice.
Serve immediately over ice, if desired.

GREEK YOGURT WITH MIXED BERRIES
Ingredients:
1 cup Greek yogurt
1/2 cup mixed berries (such as strawberries, blueberries, raspberries)
Instructions:
Spoon Greek yogurt into a bowl or serving dish.
Top the yogurt with a variety of mixed berries.
Gently mix the berries into the yogurt if desired.
Enjoy the creamy Greek yogurt with mixed berries as a nutritious and refreshing snack or breakfast option.

SLICED CUCUMBER WITH TZATZIKI SAUCE
Ingredients:
1 cucumber, sliced
1/4 cup tzatziki sauce
Instructions:
Wash the cucumber and slice it into thin rounds or sticks.
Arrange the cucumber slices on a plate or serving dish.
Serve the sliced cucumber with a side of tzatziki sauce for dipping.
Enjoy the crisp and cool cucumber slices with creamy tzatziki sauce as a light and refreshing snack.

TRAIL MIX WITH NUTS AND DRIED FRUIT
Ingredients:
1/2 cup mixed nuts (such as almonds, walnuts, cashews)
1/4 cup dried fruit (such as raisins, cranberries, apricots)
Optional: dark chocolate chips or seeds (such as pumpkin seeds)
Instructions:
In a bowl, combine the mixed nuts, dried fruit, and any optional ingredients.
Mix well to distribute the ingredients evenly.
Transfer the trail mix to a resealable container or portion into individual snack bags for on-the-go convenience.
Enjoy the trail mix.

EDAMAME
Ingredients:
1 cup edamame (shelled)
Instructions:
Bring a pot of water to a boil.
Add the edamame to the boiling water and cook for about 5-7 minutes or until tender.
Drain the edamame and rinse with cold water.
Serve the edamame as a healthy snack, either warm or chilled.

OAT BERRY SMOOTHIE
Ingredients:
1/2 cup rolled oats
1 cup mixed berries (such as strawberries,
blueberries, raspberries)
1 ripe banana
1 cup almond milk (or any milk of your choice)
1 tablespoon honey or maple syrup (optional)
1/2 teaspoon vanilla extract
Ice cubes (optional)
Instructions:
In a blender, add the rolled oats and blend until they
become a fine powder.
Add the mixed berries, ripe banana, almond milk,
honey or maple syrup (if using), and vanilla extract
to the blender.
Blend until smooth and well combined. If desired,
add a few ice cubes to make the smoothie colder.
Pour the smoothie into a glass and serve
immediately.

OATMEAL MUFFINS
Ingredients:
1 1/2 cups all-purpose flour
1 cup old-fashioned rolled oats
1/2 cup brown sugar
2 tsp baking powder
1/2 tsp baking soda
1/2 tsp salt

1 cup milk
1/4 cup vegetable oil
1 egg
1 tsp vanilla extract
Instructions:
Preheat the oven to 375°F.
In a large bowl, whisk together flour, rolled oats,
brown sugar, baking powder, baking soda, and salt.
In a separate bowl, whisk together milk, vegetable
oil, egg, and vanilla extract.
Pour wet ingredients into dry ingredients and mix
until just combined.
Pour batter into lined muffin tins, filling each cup
about 3/4 full.
Bake for 20-25 minutes, until muffins are golden
brown and a toothpick inserted into the center
comes out clean.
Allow muffins to cool in the tin for 5 minutes
before removing and transferring to a wire rack to
cool completely.

ZUCCHINI MUFFINS
Ingredients:
1 1/2 cups all-purpose flour
1/2 cup whole wheat flour
1/2 cup granulated sugar
2 tsp baking powder
1 tsp ground cinnamon
1/2 tsp salt

2 eggs
1/2 cup unsweetened applesauce
1/4 cup vegetable oil
1 tsp vanilla extract
1 1/2 cups grated zucchini (about 2 small zucchinis)
1/2 cup chopped walnuts (optional)
Instructions:
Preheat the oven to 375°F.

In a large bowl, whisk together flours, sugar, baking powder, cinnamon, and salt.

In a separate bowl, whisk together eggs, applesauce, vegetable oil, and vanilla extract.

Pour wet ingredients into dry ingredients and mix until just combined.

Fold in grated zucchini and chopped walnuts, if using.

Pour batter into lined muffin tins, filling each cup about 3/4 full.

Bake for 25-30 minutes, until muffins are golden brown and a toothpick inserted into the center comes out clean.

Allow muffins to cool in the tin for 5 minutes before removing and transferring to a wire rack to cool completely.

RASPBERRY CHIA PUDDING
Ingredients:
1/4 cup chia seeds
1 cup almond milk (or any milk of your choice)
1 tablespoon honey or maple syrup
1/2 teaspoon vanilla extract
1/2 cup fresh raspberries
Optional toppings: additional fresh raspberries, sliced almonds, or shredded coconut
Instructions:
In a bowl, combine the chia seeds, almond milk, honey or maple syrup, and vanilla extract. Stir well to combine.
Let the mixture sit for about 5 minutes, then give it another stir to prevent clumping.
Cover the bowl and place it in the refrigerator for at least 2 hours, or overnight, to allow the chia seeds to absorb the liquid and thicken.
Once the chia pudding has set, give it a good stir to break up any clumps.
Divide the pudding into serving bowls or glasses.
Top the pudding with fresh raspberries and any optional toppings you desire, such as sliced almonds or shredded coconut.
Serve and enjoy.

CITRUS BEET JUICE

Ingredients:
1 medium beet, peeled and chopped
2 apples, cored and chopped
1 orange, peeled and segmented
1 lemon, juiced
1-inch piece of ginger, peeled
Optional: honey or maple syrup for sweetness

Instructions:
Place the chopped beet, apples, orange segments, lemon juice, and ginger in a juicer.
Process the ingredients until they are well juiced and combined.
Taste the juice and add a small amount of honey or maple syrup if desired for added sweetness.
Stir the juice well to incorporate the sweetener.
Pour the apple and citrus beet juice into glasses and serve immediately.
Enjoy the refreshing and nutritious juice as a morning pick-me-up or as a healthy beverage throughout the day.

APPLE SLICES WITH ALMOND BUTTER

Ingredients:
1 apple (any variety), sliced
2 tablespoons almond butter

Instructions:
Wash and core the apple, then slice it into thin rounds or wedges.

Spread almond butter on one side of each apple slice.

Arrange the apple slices on a plate or serving dish.
Serve the apple slices with almond butter as a healthy and satisfying snack.

CARROT STICKS WITH HUMMUS
Ingredients:
2 carrots, peeled and cut into sticks
1/4 cup hummus
Instructions:
Peel the carrots and cut them into long, thin sticks.
Place the carrot sticks on a plate or serving dish.
Serve the carrot sticks with a side of hummus for dipping.
Enjoy the crunchy and nutritious carrot sticks with creamy hummus as a delicious snack.

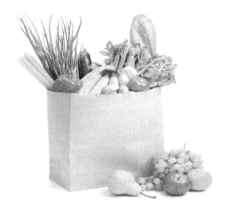

Dear Friend,

I hope this letter finds you in good health and high spirits. I wanted to take a moment to express my heartfelt gratitude for your purchase of the Ornish Diet cookbook. Your support not only encourages me as an author but also contributes to spreading the message of healthy living and nourishing our bodies through mindful eating.

Thank you for choosing the Ornish Diet cookbook as your guide to a healthier lifestyle. By investing in this book, you have taken a proactive step towards improving your well-being and embracing a diet that promotes vitality and heart health. I am truly honored to be a part of your journey.

I want to assure you that every recipe has been meticulously tested and developed with utmost care. My aim was to create a collection that not only offers a variety of flavors but also makes it easy for you to incorporate the Ornish Diet into your daily routine. It is my hope that these recipes will inspire you to experiment, enjoy the process of cooking, and discover the immense pleasure in nourishing yourself and your loved ones.

As you embark on this culinary adventure, I encourage you to remember the importance of balance and self-care. In these challenging times, I would like to extend my warmest wishes for your continued health and safety. Please take care of yourself and your loved ones, and remember to embrace joy, gratitude, and the simple pleasures that life offers.

Once again, thank you for choosing the Ornish Diet cookbook. Your support means the world to me, and I hope this book becomes a trusted companion on your journey towards a healthier and more fulfilling life.

Stay safe and healthy, and may your culinary endeavors be filled with delight and nourishment.

With sincere appreciation,
Curnow K. Rivers

CONCLUSION

In conclusion, the ORNISH diet cookbook is a useful tool for anyone wishing to adopt a healthier way of life and enhance their general well-being. Individuals might achieve great improvements in their overall health by adhering to the ORNISH diet's tenets. The meticulously chosen assortment of meals in this cookbook demonstrates the amazing variety and delectability that may be attained while adhering to the ORNISH diet requirements.

The ORNISH diet supports heart health, weight control, and avoiding illnesses through the use of nutrient-dense, plant-based components. It also nourishes the body. Lean foods, fruits, veggies, legumes, and whole grains can all be found in our meals to help us take charge of our health and achieve lifelong improvements.

This cookbook equips people to make flavorful and satisfying meals that adhere to the ORNISH diet guidelines by carefully crafting each recipe and including comprehensive instructions. The recipes provided here offer a wide range of options for every palate, from robust breakfasts to filling lunches and delicious feasts.

You can start along the path to better health, vigor, and longevity by adopting the ORNISH diet and using the recipes in this cookbook. In order to learn the delight of nourishing your body and enjoying delectable meals that promote your well-being, let this cookbook serve as your guide. Begin your culinary journey right away and discover the ORNISH diet's transformational potential.

14 DAY MEAL PLAN

Day 1:
Breakfast: Blueberry Oatmeal Bowl with Almond Milk and Chia Seeds
Lunch: Quinoa and Chickpea Salad with Lemon-Tahini Dressing
Snack: Fresh Fruit Salad
Dinner: Lentil Bolognese over Whole Wheat Spaghetti
Dessert: Baked Apples with Cinnamon and Walnuts
Day 2:
Breakfast: Spinach and Mushroom Tofu Scramble
Lunch: Black Bean and Corn Salad with Avocado Dressing
Snack: Carrot Sticks with Hummus
Dinner: Stuffed Bell Peppers with Quinoa and Black Beans
Dessert: Chocolate Chia Pudding
Day 3:
Breakfast: Banana Walnut Pancakes with Maple Syrup
Lunch: Mediterranean Couscous Salad with Roasted Vegetables
Snack: Trail Mix with Nuts and Dried Fruits
Dinner: Eggplant Rollatini with Tofu Ricotta
Dessert: Mixed Berry Parfait with Coconut Yogurt
Day 4:
Breakfast: Overnight Chia Pudding with Mixed Berries
Lunch: Lentil and Vegetable Curry with Brown Rice
Snack: Edamame Beans
Dinner: Sweet Potato and Black Bean Enchiladas
Dessert: Coconut Mango Sorbet
Day 5:
Breakfast: Green Smoothie Bowl with Spinach, Banana, and Almond Milk
Lunch: Quinoa and Roasted Vegetable Buddha Bowl with Tahini Dressing
Snack: Roasted Chickpeas

Dinner: Portobello Mushroom Burger with Sweet Potato Fries
Dessert: Vegan Chocolate Mousse
Day 6:
Breakfast: Avocado Toast with Sliced Tomatoes and Sprouts
Lunch: Greek Salad with Tofu Feta
Snack: Celery Sticks with Peanut Butter
Dinner: Ratatouille with Herbed Quinoa
Dessert: Mixed Berry Crumble
Day 7:
Breakfast: Apple Cinnamon Overnight Oats
Lunch: Roasted Vegetable Wrap with Hummus
Snack: Fresh Fruit Smoothie
Dinner: Veggie Stir-Fry with Brown Rice
Dessert: Lemon Poppy Seed Energy Balls
Day 8:
Breakfast: Vegan Protein Pancakes with Berry Compote
Lunch: Mediterranean Chickpea Salad with Cucumber and Olives
Snack: Rice Cakes with Almond Butter
Dinner: Spaghetti Squash with Marinara Sauce and Vegan Meatballs
Dessert: Mango Coconut Chia Pudding
Day 9:
Breakfast: Quinoa Breakfast Bowl with Mixed Berries and Almond Milk
Lunch: Caprese Salad with Balsamic Glaze
Snack: Kale Chips
Dinner: Vegetable Curry with Coconut Milk and Brown Rice
Dessert: Raspberry Nice Cream
Day 10:
Breakfast: Vegan Breakfast Burrito with Tofu Scramble and Black Beans
Lunch: Asian Noodle Salad with Peanut Sauce
Snack: Homemade Popcorn with Sea Salt
Dinner: Cauliflower Steak with Roasted Vegetables

Dessert: Matcha Green Tea Energy Balls

Day 11:
Breakfast: Mixed Berry Smoothie Bowl with Granola Topping
Lunch: Quinoa and Lentil Stuffed Bell Peppers
Snack: Sliced Bell Peppers with Hummus
Dinner: Zucchini Noodles with Creamy Avocado Pesto
Dessert: Banana Ice Cream with Almond Butter Drizzle

Day 12:
Breakfast: Vegan French Toast with Fresh Berries
Lunch: Mediterranean Hummus Wrap with Veggies
Snack: Ants on a Log (Celery with Peanut Butter and Raisins)
Dinner: Portobello Mushroom Fajitas with Whole Wheat Tortillas
Dessert: Coconut Lime Chia Pudding

Day 13:
Breakfast: Green Smoothie with Spinach, Pineapple, and Coconut Water
Lunch: Quinoa and Chickpea Stuffed Sweet Potato
Snack: Roasted Almonds
Dinner: Lentil and Vegetable Stir-Fry with Brown Rice
Dessert: Vegan Chocolate Chip Cookies

Day 14:
Breakfast: Acai Bowl with Mixed Fruit and Granola Topping
Lunch: Greek Quinoa Salad with Tofu Skewers
Snack: Veggie Crudité with Hummus
Dinner: Vegan Mushroom Risotto
Dessert: Mixed Berry Cobbler

STAY SAFE AND HEALTHY

WEEKLY MEAL PLANNER

			GROCERY LIST
MONDAY	BREAKFAST		
	LUNCH		
	DINNER		
TUESDAY	BREAKFAST		
	LUNCH		
	DINNER		
WEDNESDAY	BREAKFAST		
	LUNCH		
	DINNER		
THURSDAY	BREAKFAST		
	LUNCH		
	DINNER		
FRIDAY	BREAKFAST		
	LUNCH		SNACKS
	DINNER		
SATURDAY	BREAKFAST		
	LUNCH		
	DINNER		
SUNDAY	BREAKFAST		
	LUNCH		
	DINNER		

WEEKLY MEAL PLANNER

			GROCERY LIST
MONDAY	BREAKFAST		
	LUNCH		
	DINNER		
TUESDAY	BREAKFAST		
	LUNCH		
	DINNER		
WEDNESDAY	BREAKFAST		
	LUNCH		
	DINNER		
THURSDAY	BREAKFAST		
	LUNCH		
	DINNER		
FRIDAY	BREAKFAST		
	LUNCH		SNACKS
	DINNER		
SATURDAY	BREAKFAST		
	LUNCH		
	DINNER		
SUNDAY	BREAKFAST		
	LUNCH		
	DINNER		

WEEKLY MEAL PLANNER

			GROCERY LIST
MONDAY	BREAKFAST		
	LUNCH		
	DINNER		
TUESDAY	BREAKFAST		
	LUNCH		
	DINNER		
WEDNESDAY	BREAKFAST		
	LUNCH		
	DINNER		
THURSDAY	BREAKFAST		
	LUNCH		
	DINNER		
FRIDAY	BREAKFAST		SNACKS
	LUNCH		
	DINNER		
SATURDAY	BREAKFAST		
	LUNCH		
	DINNER		
SUNDAY	BREAKFAST		
	LUNCH		
	DINNER		

WEEKLY MEAL PLANNER

			GROCERY LIST
MONDAY	BREAKFAST		
	LUNCH		
	DINNER		
TUESDAY	BREAKFAST		
	LUNCH		
	DINNER		
WEDNESDAY	BREAKFAST		
	LUNCH		
	DINNER		
THURSDAY	BREAKFAST		
	LUNCH		
	DINNER		
FRIDAY	BREAKFAST		SNACKS
	LUNCH		
	DINNER		
SATURDAY	BREAKFAST		
	LUNCH		
	DINNER		
SUNDAY	BREAKFAST		
	LUNCH		
	DINNER		

Made in United States
North Haven, CT
08 November 2024